Keto Diet Guide
Create Your Own Lifestyle

With

30 Easy Delicious Keto Diet Recipes with Nutrition Facts for Fast Lose Weight and Healthy Living in Your Own Keto Diet Lifestyle

Table Of Contents

Introduction 1

Chapter 1: What is a Ketogenic Diet? 3

Chapter 2: What Types of Foods to Choose 12

Chapter 3: How to Avoid the Keto Flu 20

Chapter 4: A Day in the Keto Life.................................. 25

Chapter 5: Recipes.. 31

Keto-Friendly Foods Nutrition Guide 69

Conclusion 79

Introduction

Here, you will find something amazing!

If you've found this book, you're probably interested in becoming healthier. Perhaps you want to lose weight and have the body that fits your weight ideal. Maybe you have type 2 diabetes, insulin resistance, or polycystic ovary syndrome. It could be that you'd like to start burning fat instead of storing it and use your newfound energy to live your best life.

Or maybe you are curious. No matter what, welcome to a whole new world of eating, and congratulations on your first steps to a healthy, long, fulfilling life.

The ketogenic diet is a diet that heals, nourishes, and optimizes the brain and body performance. It's a natural, healthy way of eating that allows you to eat yummy foods without sacrificing satiety.

Yes, you did read that right!

You don't have to be hungry.

I didn't believe it either. Seven months ago, I was morbidly obese, bursting out of my jeans, and suffering from incredibly low self-esteem because I just didn't enjoy living in the body I had.

Today, I have lost 20% of my body weight (50 pounds!), several pants sizes, and being constantly obsessed over food. I'm in excellent health both mentally and physically, and I attribute my improved mental health to the keto diet's positive effects on my self-esteem.

The ketogenic diet has changed my relationship with food. I choose to eat to fuel my body, and in return, my body rewards me with high performance, excellent sleep, and weight loss.

So strap in and prepare to learn what the keto diet is all about, how you can get started, and which foods to make and eat to hack your fun, delicious weight-loss journey. In this e-book, I'll share the science, the protocol, and my own tried-and-true recipes that are easy to make and eat and oh so satisfying.

Welcome to the best part of your life.

Chapter 1: What is a Ketogenic Diet?

The Basics

A ketogenic diet is a high-fat, moderate protein, low-carb diet. You eat about 70% of your calories from fat, 25% from protein, and 5% from net carbohydrates. Net carbohydrates are calculated by taking the number of carbohydrates you consume and subtracting the number of grams of fiber; fiber does not raise blood sugar.

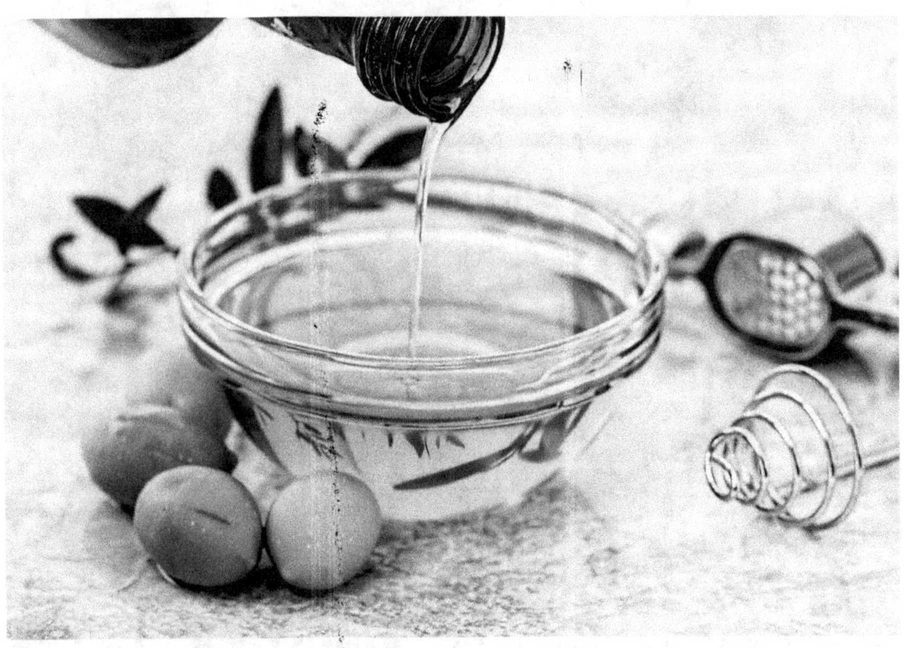

This diet is rich in whole foods like dairy, meats, and vegetables. Processed food is kept to a minimum, although you would be surprised at how many convenience foods are keto-friendly!

Essentially, the keto diet is all about keeping your blood sugar from fluctuating dramatically. This has the effect of allowing your body to concentrate on burning stored fat and operating at top efficiency. Many people who do not need to lose weight eat a ketogenic diet because of its health benefits and its ability to control blood sugar.

The Science

> **Ketosis: a state in which your body no longer runs on sugar and instead burns both consumed and stored fat.**

Ketosis

The keto diet is a diet that puts your body in a state called *ketosis*. While this might sound complicated and artificial, ketosis is a natural, healing process. As humans, we are born in a state of ketosis when we leave our mothers' bodies.

Ketosis is when your body burns ketones instead of glucose. Glucose is sugar that is found in fruit, grains, starches, sugar, and other foods.

Ketones are made in the brain when the body doesn't have glucose to burn and instead starts burning fat. It begins with fats you have eaten, and when there are no more of those to digest, your body starts burning stored body fat.

Blood sugar

Because the keto diet is so low in sugar and carbs (which are converted to sugar), your blood sugar remains steady. Your insulin doesn't have nearly as many peaks and valleys as it does on a high-carbohydrate diet; because the keto diet is so satisfying, you won't be spiking your blood sugar every couple of hours with sugar and snacks.

Diuretic Effects

Another benefit of the ketogenic diet is that it is a diuretic diet, meaning that you do not retain nearly as much water as you would on a standard diet. Carbohydrates hold onto water. Some of our excess carbs are stored as an energy reserve called glycogen in the muscles and liver, and they hold onto water there. When in ketosis, these reserves are burned and never restored, meaning that all of that excess water is no longer retained. If you have issues with swelling from water retention, the keto diet may be a good fit for you.

Cholesterol and Fat Vilification

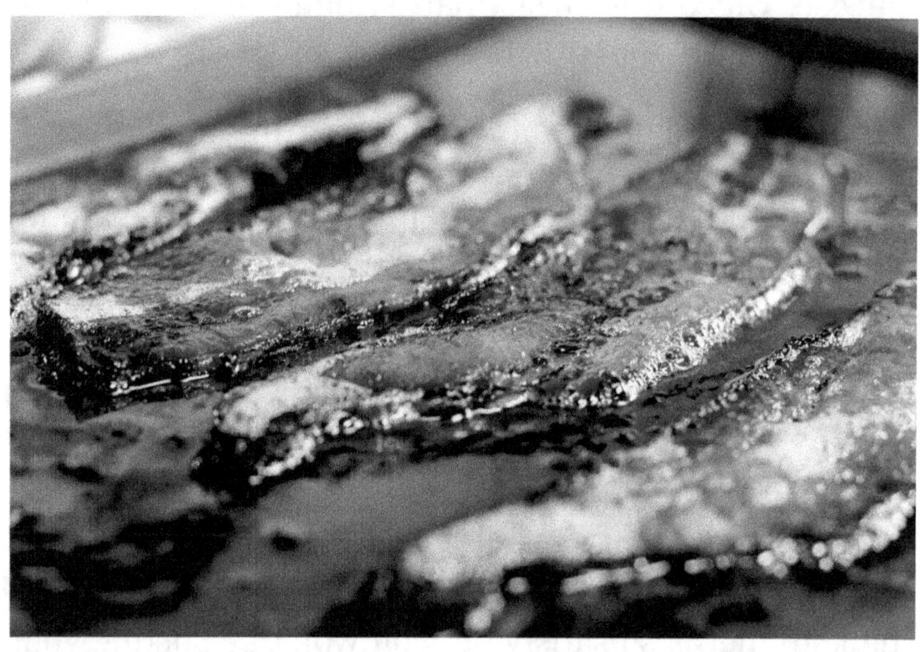

Some people may be worried about eating 70% of their calories from fat. Think of it: butter, bacon, heavy cream, fatty hamburgers, cheese... These are the foods that are supposed to clog your arteries and send you to an early grave! They're supposed to raise your cholesterol and cause problems, especially in your heart.

But the cholesterol you eat doesn't necessarily translate to your blood cholesterol. Genetic factors play a much larger role, and even the ongoing Framingham heart study, one of the first studies that led scientists to call for people to eat less dietary cholesterol, hasn't shown that the cholesterol we eat significantly raises the cholesterol that clogs our arteries.

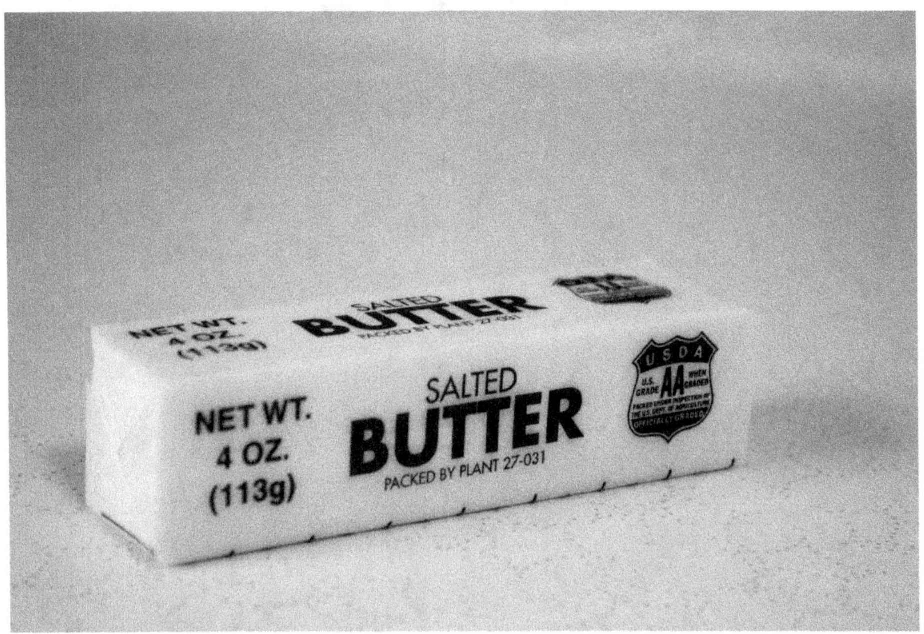

People always like to talk about how bad low-carb diets are for people, but every other week there's a success story floating around about someone who lost weight and got healthier with keto, Atkins, or South Beach.

The moral here is to take conventional dietary wisdom with a grain of salt-or more! (We'll get to sodium when we talk about electrolytes later.)

The Protocol

Keto Macros

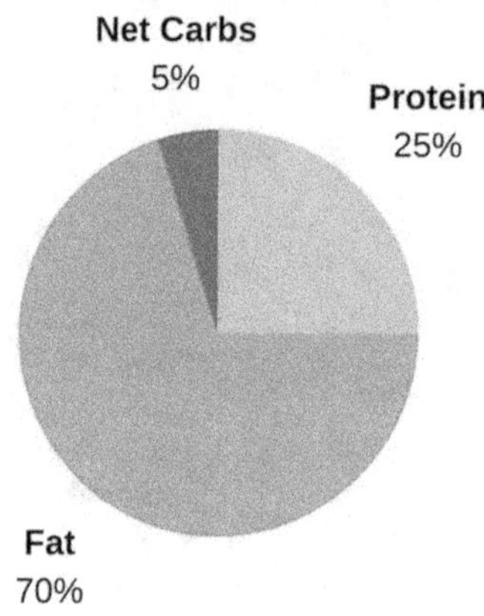

Macros

Calculating your macros

Okay, so keto is high-fat, moderate protein, low-carb, and won't kill me, you may be thinking. *What's next?*

Next, we calculate your macros.

Macronutrients are carbs, protein, and fat. They're the building blocks of food.

A standard American/Western civilization diet usually contains about 50% calories from carbs, 34% calories from fat, and 16% calories from protein.

We're going to take your diet and mess with your macros until they match roughly 70% fat, 25% protein, and 5% carbs.

It's important to note that everyone's macronutrient goals are going to be different. Lots of things factor into the optimal eating plan for each person.

Also, in weight loss mode, some of the 70% of energy from fats ***comes from stored fat***. So you might not be EATING 70% fat, but 70% of your body's energy comes from fat.

Gender, age, weight, height, activity level, body fat percentage, and other factors all contribute to a person's macros.

For example, a 22-year-old woman who is 5'4", weighs 205 pounds, has 40% body fat, and wants to eat at a 25% calorie deficit while maintaining muscle mass has the following macronutrient and calorie goals:
1570 calories
109g fats
25g carbs
123g protein.

As stated above, these macros are not perfect 70/25/5 macros, and this is perfectly okay.

In contrast, a 35-year-old man who is 5'10", weighs 300 lbs, has 35% body fat and wants to eat at a 20% calorie deficit while maintaining muscle mass has these macros:
2302 calories

158g fats
25g carbs
195g protein.

To calculate your own macros, simply do an internet search for **keto macro calculator.** A popular choice is made by the company Ruled.Me.

Tracking your macros

To keep track of how much you're actually eating, you have two main options:

- Go old-fashioned! Read nutrition labels and write down the macro information from your foods in a notebook. Keep a daily tally.
- Embrace the convenience of apps. Popular apps include MyFitnessPal, SparkPeople, Cronometer, and Carb Manager. Many of these are free!

"Lazy" Keto

If, *and only if*, you do not do well, counting calories or if you have suffered from an eating disorder, you may consider not tracking your macros, but instead sticking to only keto-approved foods and monitoring your carbohydrate intake.

This is not as effective as tracking your macros and there is a danger of overeating. However, many people find weight loss success through lazy keto simply because they are not eating as much due to the satiation effect of high-fat, low-carb living.

Chapter 2: What Types of Foods to Choose

Keto may seem daunting just because of the carbohydrate-rich foods you will be choosing not to have. However, there are many types of delicious foods that are keto-friendly. For a nutrition list of several basic keto-friendly foods, see the Appendix to this book. For now, here are some types of foods that will give you delicious, satisfying meals.

Meat & Fish

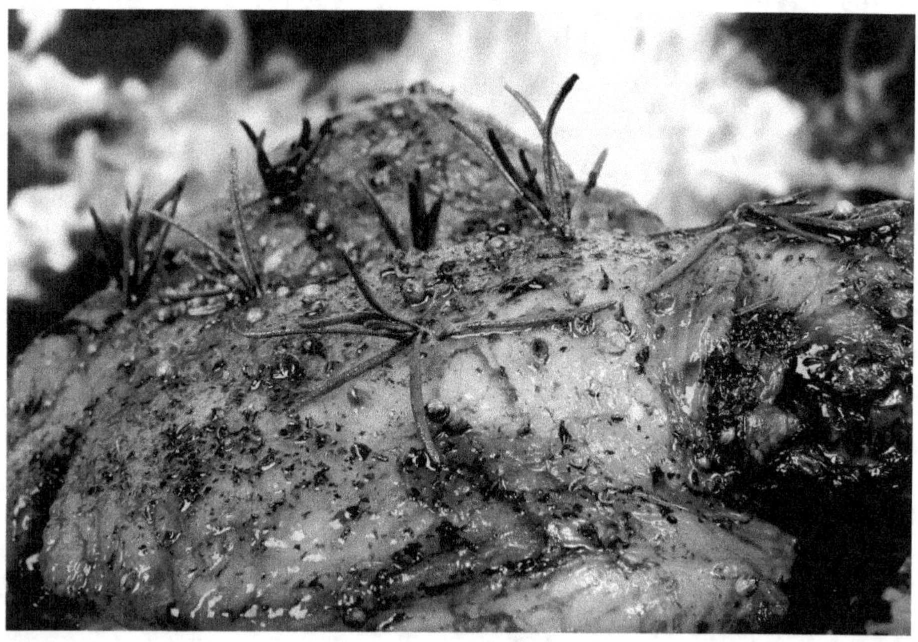

Any meat that is not sweetened with sugar or flavored with carbohydrates is acceptable to a keto way of life. The fattier the meat, the better! Remember that breading contains carbohydrates, so choose grilled, baked, broiled, or sauteed meats. Popular choices include:
- Beef:
  - Fatty hamburger

- ○ Chuck roast
- ○ Steaks like New York strip, ribeye, and t-bone cuts
- ○ Corned beef brisket
- Poultry (skin-on)
  - ○ Chicken (all parts)
  - ○ Turkey (all parts)
- Pork
  - ○ Ribs
  - ○ Shoulder roast
  - ○ Bacon
- Fish
  - ○ Salmon
  - ○ Mackerel
  - ○ Tuna

Vegetables

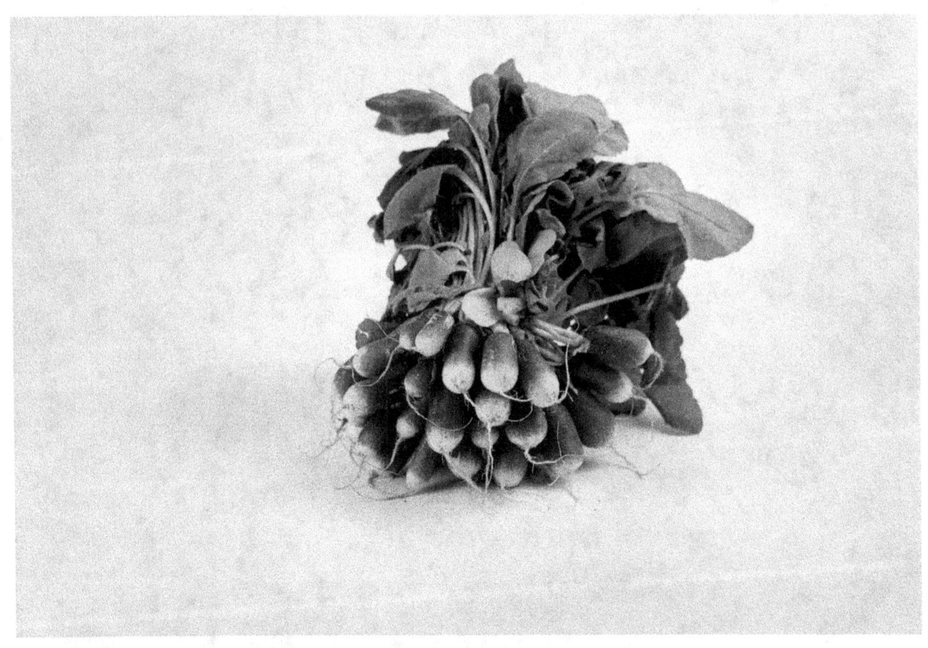

Vegetables do contain carbohydrates. However, they should be your preferred source of carbohydrates because they contain fiber, which is not processed as a carb by the body. Instead, fiber slows the absorption of carbohydrates and helps mitigate bad blood sugar effects. In addition, you need vitamins and minerals that are found in vegetables.

- Avocado (technically a fruit)
- Cauliflower
- Zucchini
- Spinach
- Broccoli
- Asparagus
- Celery
- Kale
- Green beans

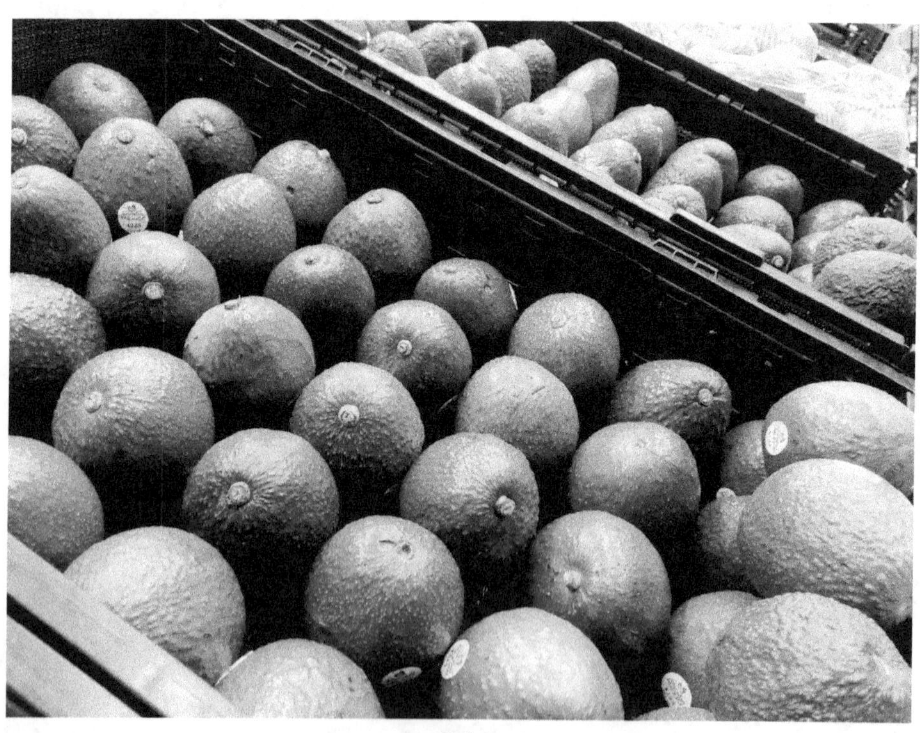

Fruit

Most fruits are a bad idea during the keto diet because the fruit is naturally very high in sugar and carbs. In small quantities, however, you can enjoy:
- Raspberries
- Blueberries
- Strawberries
- Blackberries
- Lemons
- Limes

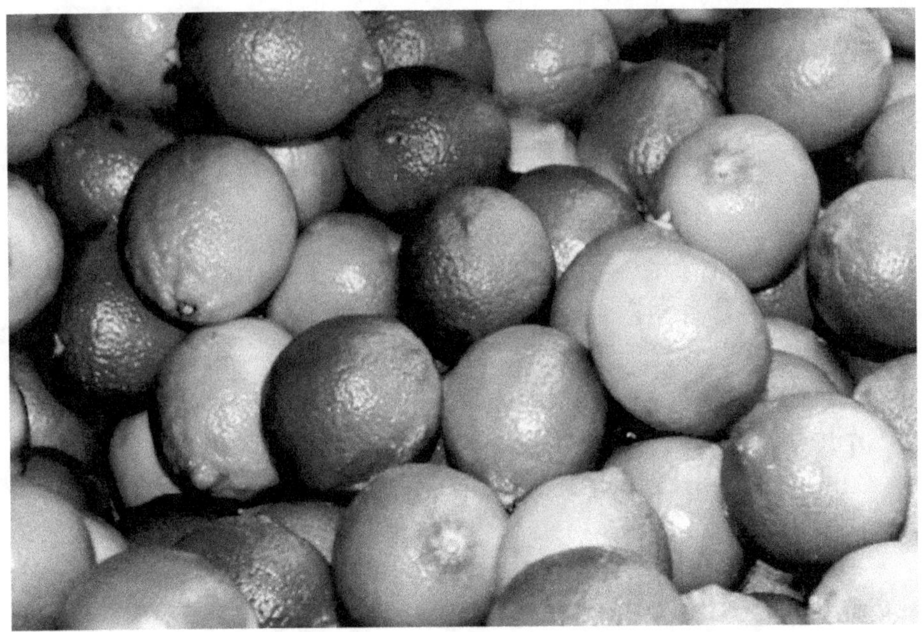

Dairy

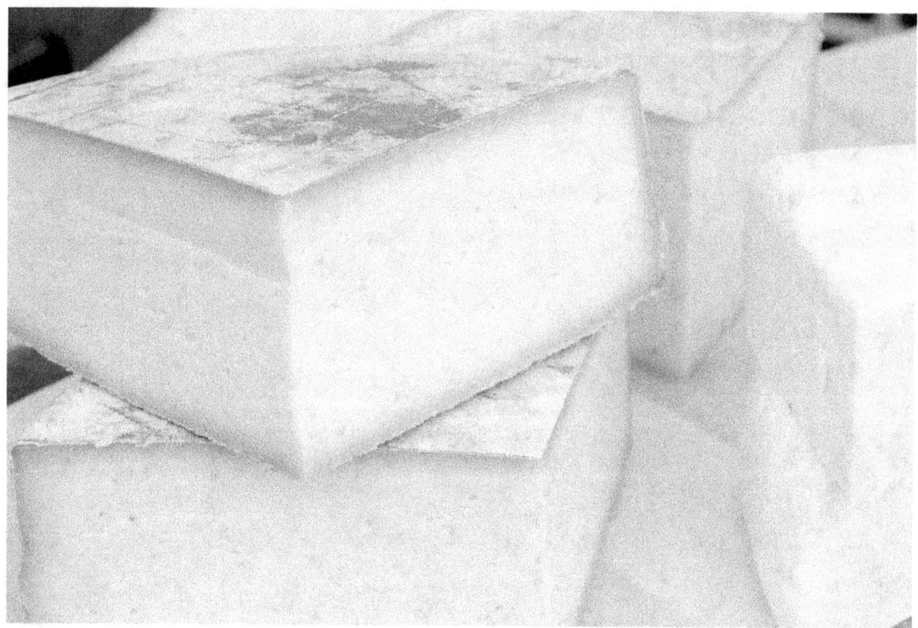

Unless you have a dairy allergy or sensitivity, you can enjoy a great deal of full-fat, delicious dairy. Choose full-fat varieties and always be mindful of carbohydrates, especially if you're looking at yogurt or milk. Many keto people stay away from plain milk because it is very high in carbohydrates. Some dairy to include in your diet is:

- Butter
- Heavy whipping cream
- Shredded cheeses (all types)
- Block cheeses
- Cream cheese
- Cottage cheese

Nuts and Seeds & Their Products

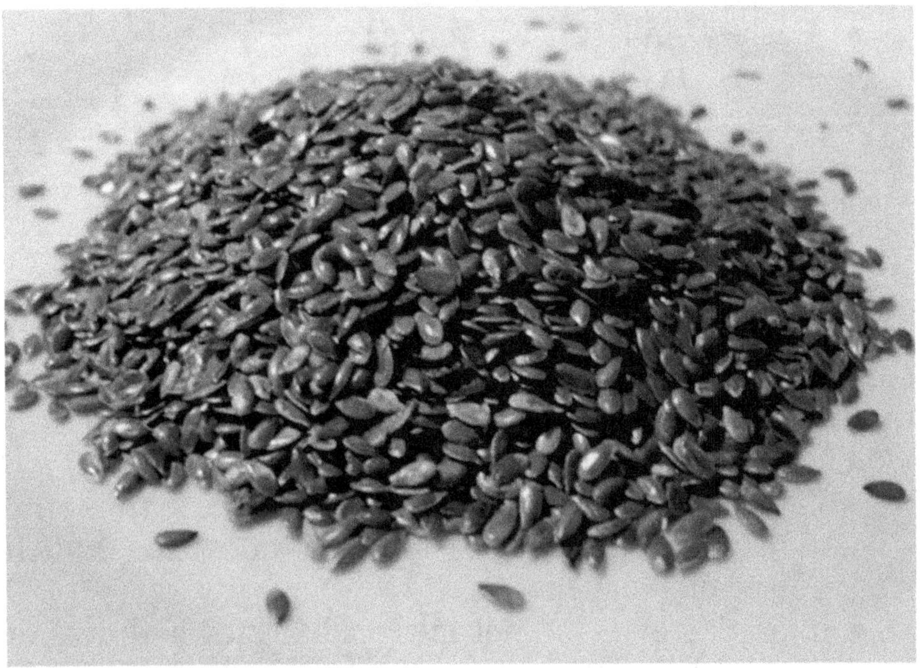

Nuts and seeds are great sources of fat! Choose nuts that are lower in carbs and remember that peanuts are actually a legume, so they tend to be higher in carbs. Some favorite nuts and nut products are:
- Almonds
- Almond meal
- Almond flour
- Coconut (unsweetened)
- Coconut flour
- Macadamia nuts
- Pecans
- Walnuts
- Cashews (be careful with these as they are higher in carbs)
- Almond butter (no sugar added)

- Peanut butter (no sugar added)
- Almond milk (unsweetened)
- Cashew milk (unsweetened)
- Flaxseed (whole or ground)
- Chia seeds (whole or ground)

Sweeteners

Because sugar is so high in carbs and spikes your blood sugar, you have to avoid it. Sweetness, however, isn't something you have to give up. Here are some good options for sweeteners that are low glycemic index and won't spike your blood sugar significantly:

- Liquid sucralose as in sugar-free coffee syrups (the powdered form contains maltodextrin, which raises blood sugar!)
- Liquid stevia (sometimes called stevia drops of stevia glycerite)
- Erythritol/Swerve (a popular sugar alcohol that behaves VERY similarly to real sugar in baking and cooking)
- Xylitol (another popular sugar alcohol, but if you own pets, be very careful as this is incredibly toxic to dogs)
- Aspartame/diet sodas (these are not the healthiest choice, but drinking them in moderation is acceptable)
- Monkfruit sweeteners

Foods to avoid

With all of the healthy and delicious options you have to choose from, it's a lot easier than you think to avoid the foods below, which are all high in starches and sugar:
- Grains and grain products, including
  - Bread
  - Pasta
  - Rice
  - Corn
- Fruits not listed in this guide
- Starchy vegetables like potatoes and beans
- Regular dairy milk (it has nearly 13 grams of carbs per cup!)
- Added sugars, like
  - Honey
  - Cane sugar
  - Maltose
  - Dextrose
  - Maltodextrin
  - Agave nectar
  - Corn syrup

A general rule of thumb is to **read the nutrition facts and avoid anything high in carbohydrates. Many proponents of the keto diet swear by never going over 20 grams of net carbs, regardless of whether their macros allow it.**

Chapter 3: How to Avoid the Keto Flu

If you do any research at all into a keto diet, you'll begin to see accounts of the "keto flu," a condition which strikes anywhere from 1-3 days into the diet and can last for a week or so. Victims complain of headaches, grumpiness, brain fog, aches, twitchiness, trouble sleeping, and a general sense of malaise. This is also called the low-carb flu and is common with any diet that has the participant abruptly switch to an ultra-low carb lifestyle.

Drink Water!

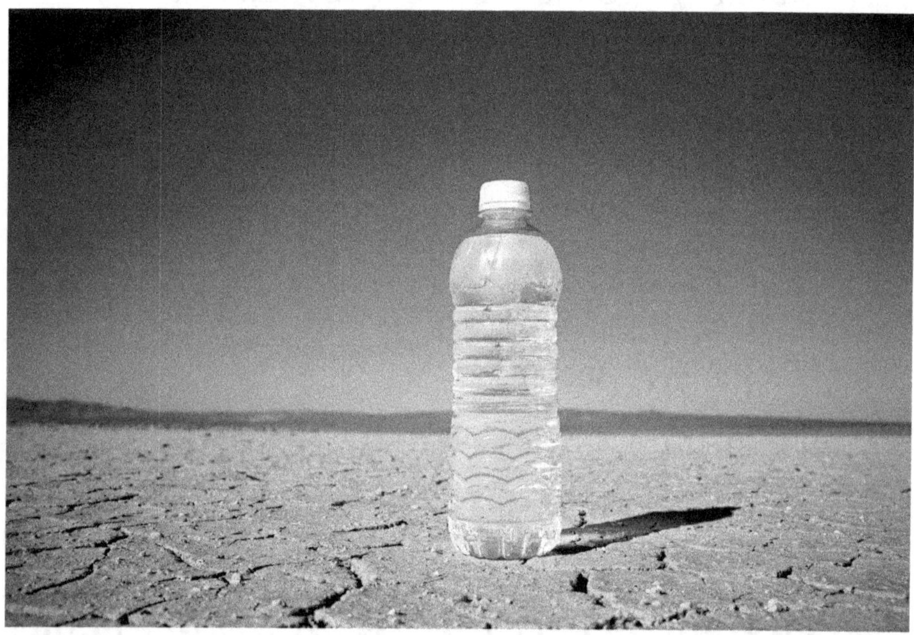

As mentioned above in Chapter 2, the keto diet has a diuretic effect. When the body doesn't hold onto excess water, it eliminates it through urine. This means that you have less water available in your body for it to use, so you need to be sipping on water all day in order to make sure that you're fully hydrated. Camels have big humps on their backs so they can store water and go a long time without drinking. Think of yourself as a camel who has relieved herself of the heavy burden on her back. You feel a lot lighter and look a lot thinner, but you need to remember to hydrate more often to offset these benefits.

Another issue is that other things are also flushed out with the water: namely, electrolytes.

Get Your Electrolytes!

Daily Electrolytes for Keto

Sodium: 5000-7000mg

Potassium: 1000-3500mg

Magnesium: 300-500mg (best before bed)

The three electrolytes that you have to worry about depleting through a regular ketogenic diet are sodium, magnesium, and potassium. These are all very important for your cells to perform their basic functions, so it's vital to keep track of these. You can track them through apps like MyFitnessPal.

On a ketogenic diet, you're going to need more of these electrolytes than your standard American diet counterparts.

The image above shows the approximate amounts you will need. It's entirely possible to get these through food, although many people find that it is easier to take supplements than to worry about eating a minimum amount of spinach every day. Supplementing is easy to do!

Magnesium supplements are available in the vitamin aisle of most grocery stores and pharmacies. Take one tablet that is a 300-500 mg dose before bed at night. Magnesium is great for soothing anxiety and helping quiet the mind, so this is not one that you'll want to take first thing in the morning. It may quiet your mind enough to leave you dozing in your morning coffee!

Sodium and potassium are a little more difficult to supplement. Many people simply salt their food for sodium, but even then it is difficult to get enough.

One way to ensure you get all the electrolytes you need is to make a homemade electrolyte drink. While there are sugar-free electrolyte drinks available, these can be very low in electrolytes even if they are delicious.

A great alternative is to buy table salt or pink Himalayan salt and a potassium-rich salt replacement product like No-Salt or Lite Salt. Measure out ¼ teaspoon of each of these and mix it into a big glass of water. To make this more palatable, add a squeeze of lime juice and a few drops of stevia or use a sugar-free water enhancer like Crystal Lite or Mio.

Drink a couple of these throughout the day and you're well on your way to getting the electrolytes you need and avoiding the keto flu!

Eat Enough Food

There seem to be two camps of people when starting a keto diet: those who are not hungry and those who are ravenous.

If you're in the first camp, you are already benefiting from the satiating effect of fat! This is wonderful. If you are losing weight, continue eating to satisfaction. If you don't hit your calorie goal for the day, that's okay! Just try to keep your ratio as close to 70/25/5 as possible.

If you're in the second camp, don't worry! Your body is going through a big adjustment and you may be more reliant on carbs than you think. Your body is telling you to feed it because it wants glucose, not protein or fat. It hasn't yet figured ketosis out after being out of it for so long since your birth. Be patient with yourself, and if needed, eat extra calories from fat. Good options for snacks are avocados, nuts, cheeses, and fatty meats.

Regardless of how hungry you are, be patient with your body as it heals and makes sure you're not starving yourself! So long as you stay below your basic calorie needs for the day, you will be burning stored body fat.

Chapter 4: A Day in the Keto Life

You may be reading this, nodding, taking notes, and finding that your head spins with all of the information I am throwing at you.

Take a breath. It's okay! It's a lot to take in at once. Now that you know what the keto diet is, what delicious foods you'll be eating, and how to avoid feeling sick as you get acclimated to ketosis, I'll walk you through how a typical keto day works.

Breakfast

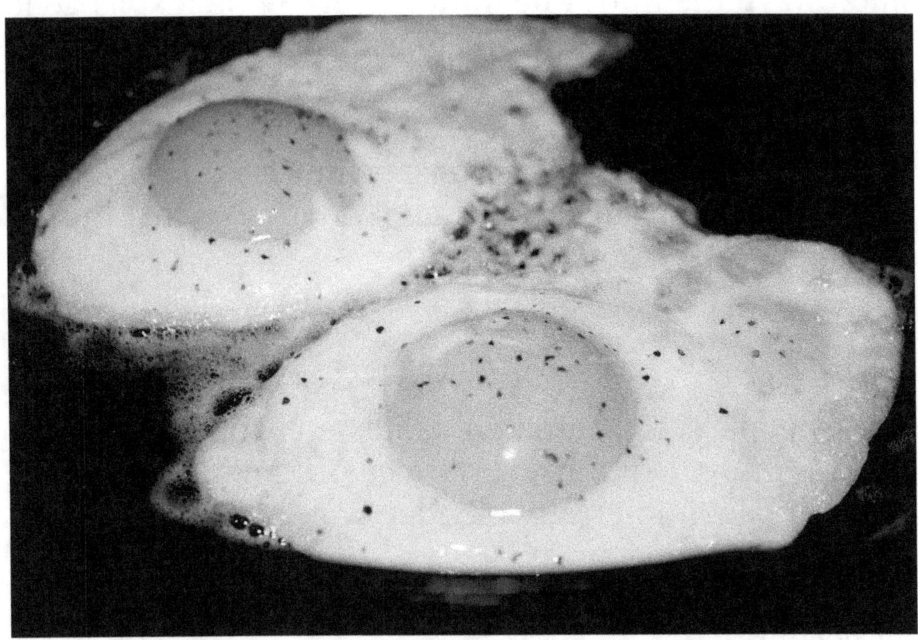

Many people on the keto diet enjoy delicious breakfasts of bacon or sausage and eggs or other high-protein, high-fat meals that require cooking. This is certainly a great option and if you enjoy a big breakfast and have the time to cook it, it's a wonderful option.

If you're like me, however, you work and don't really want to drag yourself out of bed an hour earlier just to make breakfast. At this point, you have two options:

Pre-prepped easy foods

No, I'm not talking about donuts or toaster pastries. In this cookbook, I have included two delicious muffin recipes. If you make a batch of muffins on the weekend, simply store them in the freezer in a ziplock bag. Pull however many muffins fits your macros out of the freezer, wrap them in a damp paper towel, and microwave them for one minute. They'll be just as good as fresh, and will take you all of 2 minutes from freezer to mouth.

Another quick and easy options include hard-boiled eggs, low-carb protein shakes, a couple spoonfuls of nut butter, or full-fat cottage cheese.

Butter coffee

Some people simply aren't breakfasted people, and that's okay! Simply take 8 oz of your favorite coffee, hot, and blend it (an immersion blender works great for this!) with the following:
1 T Butter
1 T coconut oil
Pinch cinnamon
Stevia drops to taste
Splash of heavy whipping cream (optional)

While butter in coffee sounds strange, it is something that many people enjoy and has the benefit of making you feel full without you actually having to consume food.

Lunch

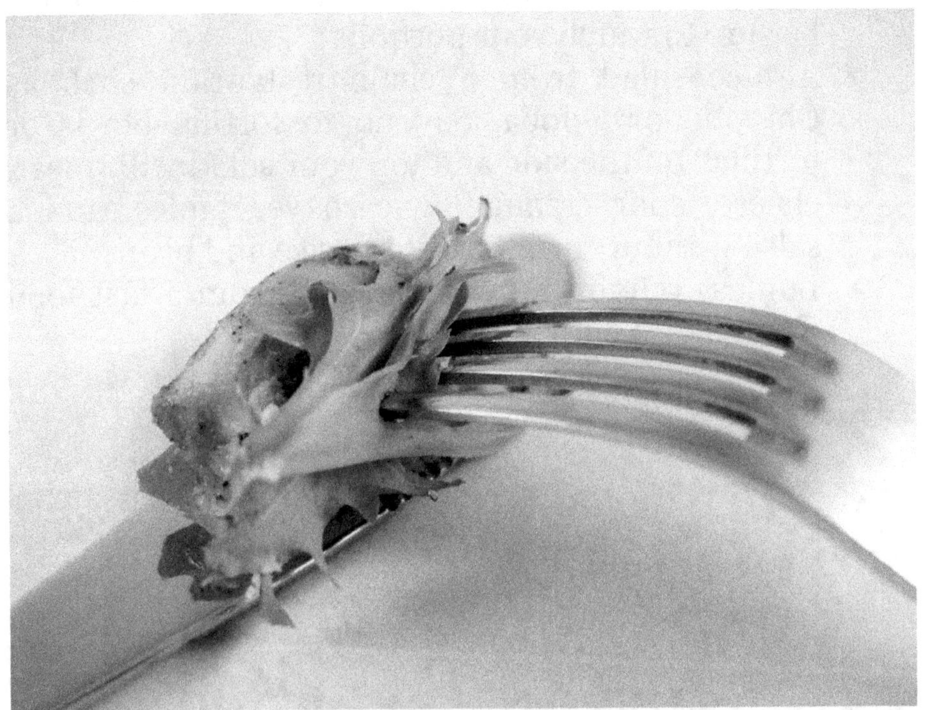

If you're a working person, you probably won't have time to stop and cook in the middle of your workday. That's okay! You can always take leftovers from last night's delicious dinner to heat up in the microwave at work, or you can enjoy some of these simple lunch ideas:

- Lunchmeat roll-ups (lunchmeat, cheese, and mustard formed into rolls. No bread, almost no carbs, and lots of flavors)
- Salad made with spinach leaves, meat, eggs, cheese, and full-fat dressing (be sure to read dressing labels to watch out for added sugars!)

- Pizza dippers (pepperoni, slices of fresh mozzarella, and a small dipping cup of low-sugar marinara sauce like the recipe I have listed in this cookbook)
- Summer sausage and cheese (simple and delicious; be sure to watch your portions)
- A taco salad from a chain restaurant such as Chipotle or Qdoba. Say no to tortilla bowls or tortillas on the side and top your salad with meat, cheese, sour cream, low-carb vegetables, and a salsa without corn. Forget the rice and beans.
- Bunless burger and a side salad from a fast food chain like Wendy's.

Dinner

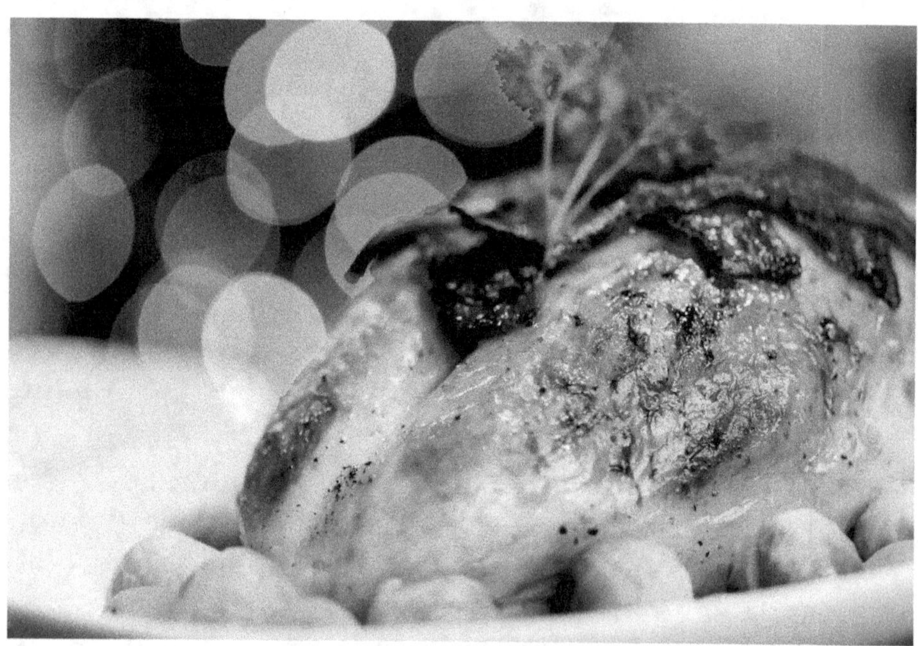

For dinner ideas, I strongly recommend trying the recipes I have included in this book! If you need to branch out, however, there are plenty of options at home or in restaurants.

At Home
To keep it simple, just build a meal with the following blocks:
- A protein (hamburger, steak, chicken, pork, beef roast, salmon, eggs, etc)
- Two low-carb vegetables (cauliflower, broccoli, zucchini, radishes, asparagus, spinach, celery)
- Butter, oil, or cheese to top the vegetables

Restaurants

Eating out is totally doable on keto! Just make sure that the ingredients are keto-approved. Popular choices include:
- Steak with a side salad and full-fat ranch dressing
- Pork chops with grilled vegetables
- Unbreaded hot wings with full-fat blue cheese or ranch dressing
- Grilled chicken or salmon with vegetables

Desserts

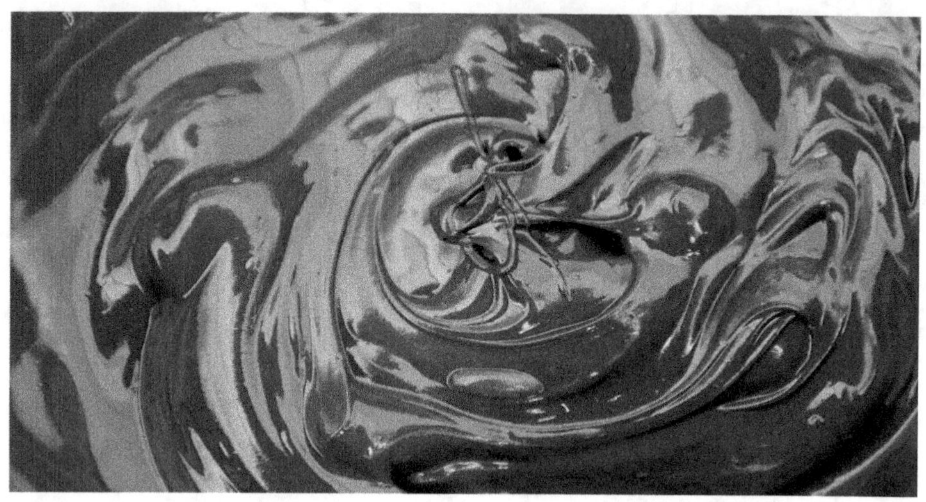

While it's best to avoid desserts if you can-even those with no added sugar-sometimes you need a little indulgence. Great options include:

- Diet soda with two tablespoons of heavy whipping cream. It takes like a soda float without all the sugar!
- Dark chocolate sweetened with stevia or erythritol
- Raspberries with homemade whipped cream sweetened with stevia or erythritol
- Cheesecake pudding (the recipe is included in this book)
- Sweet and salty cinnamon bites (the recipe is included in this book)

Now that you've got a good idea of what to eat in a day, how the keto diet works, and how to avoid common pitfalls, it's time to get cooking! The next and final chapter provides you with some tried and true recipes for delicious, nutritious weight loss.

Chapter 5: Recipes

Appetizers, Snacks & Sides

Asparagus Gratin

Ingredients

2 lbs asparagus
1 cup grated mozzarella cheese
1 cup shredded parmesan cheese
¾ cups heavy cream
3 cloves of minced garlic
Salt (¼ tsp or to taste)
Black pepper (½ tsp or to taste)

Instructions

1) Preheat oven to 400°F. Spray an 8x8 square baking dish with cooking spray.
2) Trim blunt ends of asparagus stalks, taking off about 2 inches of tough stem. Discard stems or freeze them to use for soup later.
3) Place asparagus in baking dish.
4) Mix heavy cream with garlic, salt, and pepper. Pour over asparagus.
5) Sprinkle cheeses over the top.
6) Bake for 25-30 minutes or until cheese is lightly browned and asparagus is tender.

8 servings

<u>Nutrition:</u>
Calories: 187
Carbs: 6g
Fiber: 2g
Net carbs: 4g
Protein: 11g
Fat: 14g

Buffalo Chicken Dip

Ingredients

1 block of cream cheese or Neufchatel cheese (both have the same carb count)
1 pound shredded cooked chicken (meat from a rotisserie chicken works great for this!)
½ cup Frank's Red Hot Wing Sauce
½ tsp celery salt (optional)
1 tsp black pepper
½ tsp salt
1 clove of minced garlic
1 cup shredded mild cheddar cheese
Celery, pork rinds, cheese crisps, or pepperoni chips (for serving)

Instructions

1) Preheat oven to 375° F.
2) Spray 8x8 baking dish with cooking spray.
3) In a large microwave-safe bowl, place cream cheese, buffalo sauce, celery salt, salt, pepper, and

garlic. Microwave for 1-3 minutes, stirring every 30 seconds until mixture is smooth and melted.

4) Remove bowl from microwave and add shredded chicken, stirring to combine.
5) Spread mixture into baking dish and top with shredded cheddar.
6) Bake for 25-30 minutes or until the cheese is golden brown.

8 servings

<u>Nutrition:</u>
245 calories
Carbs: 2g
Fiber: 0g
Net carbs: 2g
Protein: 22g
Fat: 17g

Beef & Cream Cheese Ball

Ingredients

1 block cream cheese or Neufchatel cheese (both have the same carb count)
5 stalks green onions
18 slices dried beef (found near the canned tuna at the grocery store)

Instructions

1) Soften cream cheese by leaving on the counter for 30 minutes. If you are in a rush, you can melt it in the microwave for about 30 seconds to soften.
2) Using kitchen shears, cut green onions into thin slices - about 1 mm wide.
3) Cut dried beef into ½ inch pieces.
4) Combine half of dried beef with all of the cream cheese and green onions. Mix well.
5) Form mixture into a ball.
6) Lay remaining dried beef on a cutting board and roll ball across it, coating the outside of the ball with dried beef.
7) Wrap in plastic wrap and chill until serving.
8) Serve on platter with a knife and desired dipping vessels (celery, pork rinds, cheese crisps, or pepperoni chips are good options)

8 servings

<u>Nutrition:</u>
Calories: 104
Carbs: 2g
Fiber: 0g
Net carbs: 2g
Protein: 3g
Fat: 10g

Cheese Crisps

Ingredients

Sandwich-style sliced Provolone cheese

Equipment
Parchment paper
Instructions

1) Cut a piece of parchment paper about the size of the rotating plate in your microwave.
2) Place 1 slice of cheese in center of parchment paper.
3) Place parchment paper in microwave and microwave for 60-90 seconds. Cheese should melt, sizzle, and turn lightly golden brown. Watch carefully so it doesn't burn.
4) Carefully remove parchment from microwave and let cool for a minute.
5) Remove crisp from parchment and break into small pieces for dipping. Repeat as desired for more crisps.

1 slice = 1 serving.

Nutrition:
Calories: 100
Carbs: 1g
Fiber: 0g
Net carbs: 1g
Protein: 7g
Fat: 8g

Garlic Mashed Cauliflower

Ingredients

1 head fresh cauliflower, cut into florets OR 1 lb frozen cauliflower florets
½ cup heavy cream
1 T cream cheese or Neufchatel cheese
2 cloves garlic
½ tsp black pepper (or to taste)
½ tsp salt (or to taste)

Instructions

1) Place a steamer insert into a saucepan and add about ½ inch of water to the bottom of the pan. Boil water and turn heat down to low. Add cauliflower, cover, and steam until tender. This usually takes about 10-15 minutes.
2) When cooked, carefully remove the cauliflower from the steamer basket and place in the bowl of a food processor.
3) Add cream, cream cheese, garlic, salt, and pepper.
4) Place lid on food processor and process until creamy.
5) If you don't have a food processor, you can use a blender or immersion blender, but you may want to add some more cream to thin the mixture out.

6 servings

<u>Nutrition:</u>
Calories: 103
Carbs: 6g
Fiber: 2g
Net carbs: 4g
Protein: 2g
Fat: 8g

Pepperoni Chips

Ingredients

Sliced pepperoni
Seasoning of choice (amount will vary based on how many chips you make. I like Cajun seasoning or Italian seasoning, but plain black pepper is also great!)

Instructions

1) Preheat oven to 375° F
2) Place pepperoni on ungreased baking sheet with sides. This is important because you don't want grease all over your oven!
3) Sprinkle with the desired seasoning or leave plain if you want to.
4) Bake for 10 minutes.
5) Remove from oven and blot away grease with paper towels.
6) Return to oven for 2-5 minutes, or until golden brown around the edges.
7) Drain on paper towels and enjoy alone or with dip! Store leftovers in a plastic bag.

16 slices of pepperoni = 1 serving

<u>Nutrition:</u>
Calories: 150
Carbs: 0
Fiber: 0
Net carbs: 0
Protein: 5g
Fat: 14g

Roasted Cauliflower & Radishes

Ingredients

1 head cauliflower
1 pound radishes
2 T lemon juice
¼ cup grated parmesan cheese
2 cloves garlic
1 tsp dried rosemary leaves
3 T olive oil
Freshly ground black pepper
Salt

Instructions

1) Preheat oven to 425° F
2) Chop cauliflower into florets
3) Wash radishes and chop off each end, then cut into quarters
4) In a medium bowl, mix lemon juice, olive oil, garlic, parmesan, and salt and pepper to taste.

5) Place chopped vegetables in a 9x13 baking dish.
6) Pour liquid mixture over the vegetables and stir to combine
7) Bake for 30 minutes, stir and then bake for an additional 15 minutes until cauliflower is golden brown around the edges and radishes are tender.

8 servings

Nutrition:
Calories: 78
Carbs: 6g
Fiber: 2g
Net carbs: 4g
Protein: 2g
Fat: 5g

Breakfast

Classic French Omelet

Ingredients

2 eggs
2 T butter
1 t water
¼ cup shredded cheese of choice
White pepper
Salt
Fresh parsley for garnish

Equipment:
Nonstick 7-inch skillet
Heat-proof rubber spatula

Instructions

1) Heat skillet over low-medium heat
2) Crack eggs into a bowl. Add water and whisk vigorously until pale yellow in color with no strings of egg white remaining, about 2-3 minutes.
3) Add salt and pepper as needed.
4) Melt 1 T of butter in heated skillet.
5) Add egg mixture to skillet.
6) Begin stirring in a figure-eight pattern, scraping down the sides. Stir constantly at a slow pace--the goal is to not allow any large curds to form.
7) Cook until eggs are set on the bottom but still slightly runny. Spread eggs out to form a single

layer in the bottom of the pan, and then sprinkle cheese on top.

8) Cook an additional 1-2 minutes or until cheese is melted.

9) Beginning at the handle of the pan, use the rubber spatula to start rolling the omelet up. Add remaining butter to the space between the omelet and the pan to make this process easier.

10)   Plate omelet and pour butter remaining in pan on the top.

11) Garnish with parsley

Variations:

Omelets are very versatile and suited for the keto lifestyle. For a larger meal, feel free to add fillings like extra cheese, cooked meats, and low-carb vegetables. A favorite of mine is cheese, avocado, and chorizo sausage.

1 serving

<u>Nutrition:</u>
Calories: 459
Carbs: 1g
Fiber: 0g
Net carbs: 1g
Protein: 20g
Fat: 42g

Lemon Poppyseed Muffins

Ingredients

1 lemon
½ cup coconut flour
4 eggs
4 T erythritol or Splenda
1 package lemon flavored sugar-free gelatine
1 T poppy seeds
1 ½ tsp baking powder
½ tsp baking soda
¼ tsp salt

Instructions

1) Preheat oven to 350° F
2) In a large bowl, combine coconut flour, sweetener, gelatine powder, baking powder, and baking soda and salt
3) Zest lemon and set the zest aside
4) Cut the lemon in half and juice it, being sure to discard the seeds.
5) In a small bowl, combine the zest and juice with the eggs. Whisk to combine.
6) Pour the egg mixture into the flour mixture and stir.
7) Add poppy seeds and stir to combine.
8) Portion out evenly into 12 paper-lined muffin cups.
9) Bake for 20-22 minutes or until a toothpick inserted in center of a muffin comes out clean.
10) Store in a sealed ziplock bag on the counter.

Tip: These freeze well. Toss the bag in the freezer. To thaw a couple of muffins, just pop them in the microwave for a minute.

12 servings.

<u>Nutrition:</u>
Calories: 124
Carbs: 3g
Fiber: 2g
Net carbs: 1g
Protein: 4g
Fat: 11g

Cinnamon Spice Oat & Flax Muffins

Ingredients

1 cup ground flax seeds
1 cup oat fiber (available on Amazon)
½ cup erythritol or Splenda
4 T melted butter
½ cup heavy whipping cream
1 T ground cinnamon
1 tsp ground cloves
1 tsp ground ginger
1 tsp baking powder
½ tsp baking soda
½ tsp vanilla extract
¼ tsp salt

Instructions

1. Preheat oven to 350° F
2. Line a muffin tin with paper liners.
3. Combine flax, oat fiber, erythritol, cinnamon, cloves, ginger, baking powder, baking soda, and salt in a large bowl.
4. In a smaller bowl, mix melted butter, cream, and vanilla.
5. Pour the contents of the smaller bowl into the larger bowl and stir well to combine. The batter will be very thick.
6. Divide evenly between 12 muffin cups and bake for 15 minutes or until a toothpick inserted in center of muffins comes out clean.

12 servings

Nutrition:
Calories: 130
Carbs: 15.4g
Fiber: 14.7g
Net carbs: 0.6g
Protein: 4g
Fat: 11g

Desserts

Cheesecake Pudding

Ingredients

1 block cream cheese or Neufchatel cheese
½ cup sour cream
½ cup heavy whipping cream
1 tsp vanilla extract
1 tsp lemon juice
½ cup Splenda OR 20 drops liquid stevia

Instructions

1) Soften cream cheese on counter OR microwave for 30 seconds.
2) In a large bowl, use a hand mixer to whip together whipping cream and sour cream until soft peaks form.
3) Add cream cheese and all other ingredients to the whipped cream mixture.
4) Whip until fully combined and fluffy.
5) Portion into 4 serving cups and chill, covered with plastic, until serving.
6) Garnish with raspberries if desired.

4 servings (6 if you add berries)

<u>Nutrition:</u>
Calories: 356
Carbs: 5g

Fiber: 0g
Net carbs: 5g
Protein: 5g
Fat: 36g

Sweet & Salty Cinnamon Bites

Ingredients

One 1.75 ounce bag of pork rinds
1 T butter
2 T erythritol or swerve
1 t cinnamon

Instructions

1) Melt butter in small bowl in the microwave
2) Place pork rinds in gallon-sized Ziploc bag
3) Pour melted butter over pork rinds
4) Add sweetener and cinnamon to the bag
5) Seal the bag
6) Shake vigorously
7) Serve immediately for a sweet and salty treat.

2 servings

Nutrition:
Calories: 177
Carbs: 2g
Fiber: 1g
Net carbs: 1g
Protein: 13g
Fat: 14g

Entrees

Braised Corned Beef

Ingredients

1 2-pound corned beef brisket
1 bottle Michelob Ultra beer or other beer with <5 grams
of carbs per bottle
2 bay leaves
5 black peppercorns

Equipment
Slow cooker

Instructions

1) Rinse corned beef under running water, making sure to save the spice packet.
2) Place corned beef in slow cooker, pouring spice mixture over top.
3) Add bay leaves and peppercorns to slow cooker.
4) Pour beer over the top of the beef. Stir.
5) Cook on low for 8 hours or on high for 4 hours. Slice and enjoy!

8 servings

Nutrition:
Calories: 210
Carbs: <1g
Fiber: 0g

Net carbs: <1g
Protein: 14g
Fat: 15g

Cajun Roast Chicken

Ingredients

4 medium chicken thighs, bone-in, skin-on
1 T Cajun seasoning
1 tsp salt (or to taste)
½ tsp pepper (or to taste)

Instructions

1) Preheat oven to 400° F.
2) Spray an 8x8 dish with cooking spray.
3) Place chicken thighs, skin-side-up, in baking dish. Sprinkle with salt, pepper, and cajun seasoning.
4) Bake uncovered for 30-35 minutes or until skin is crispy and internal temperature reaches 180° F.

4 servings

Nutrition:
Calories: 235
Carbs: 0g
Fiber: 0g
Net carbs: 0g
Protein: 23.9g
Fat: 14.7g

Cheese Crust Pizza

Ingredients

1 ½ cups shredded mozzarella cheese, divided
Pizza toppings of choice. Good options include cooked chicken, sausage, salami, pepperoni, or bacon.
Low-sugar marinara sauce (see recipe)

Equipment
Nonstick 7-inch skillet.

Instructions

1) Heat skillet over medium heat. Spray with cooking spray
2) Add 1 cup of the cheese to the skillet. Do not stir.
3) Cook until you can see the bottom of the cheese turning golden brown. The cheese will be the pizza crust, so it is important not to disturb it before it is brown.
4) Add pizza toppings to the top of the cheese, then add the rest of the cheese. Turn down to low and cover.
5) Cook until the cheese on the top is melted, then slide pizza out onto cutting board. Slice and serve with low-sugar marinara sauce for dipping.

1 serving

<u>Nutrition:</u> (just cheese - add sauce and toppings for total)
Calories: 512
Carbohydrates: 6g

Fiber: 0g
Net carbs: 6g
Protein: 44g
Fat: 34g

Easy Spiced Pot-Roast

Ingredients

1 2-pound fatty beef roast - chuck works well
6-8 pepperoncini peppers
4 T butter
1 beef bouillon cube
1 tsp garlic powder
1 T onion powder
1 T parsley flakes
2 bay leaves
Salt and pepper to taste
Xanthan gum (optional)

Equipment
Slow cooker

Instructions

1) Spray slow cooker with cooking spray OR use a plastic slow cooker liner.
2) Place roast in bottom of slow cooker.
3) Add bouillon cube, garlic powder, onion powder, parsley flakes, bay leaves, salt, and pepper.
4) Slice butter into ¼ inch pats and dot on the top of the roast.

5) Nestle pepperoncini peppers around the roast.

6) Cook on low for 8 hours or on high for 4 hours.

7) Shred with 2 forks and serve with garlic mashed cauliflower to make full use of the delicious juices.

8) If desired, add 1 tsp xanthan gum to the juices left over after you remove the roast. Whisk heavily until thickened and use as gravy.

8 servings

<u>Nutrition:</u>
Calories: 307
Carbs: 2g
Fiber: 1g
Net carbs: 1g
Protein: 20g
Fat: 24g

Lemon Thyme Chicken Thighs

Ingredients

4 chicken thighs with bones and skin intact
2 tsp smoked paprika
Salt & pepper to taste
2 T butter, divided
2 cloves minced garlic
1/2 cup chicken broth OR 1/2 cup water with 1 chicken bouillon cube dissolved in it.
¼ cup heavy whipping cream
¼ cup grated parmesan cheese
2 T lemon juice

4-5 sprigs fresh thyme OR 1 tsp dried thyme
2 cups fresh greens. I like spinach and arugula.
Instructions

1) Preheat oven to 400 F
2) Season chicken thighs paprika, salt, and pepper. Be sure to season both sides!
3) Melt 1 T butter in a cast-iron skillet or another oven-proof skillet over medium heat (If you don't have an oven-proof skillet, use a regular skillet and transfer the chicken to an 8x8 baking dish when it's time to bake it.)
4) Place chicken, skin-side down, in skillet and cook for 3-4 minutes or until golden brown. Flip and cook an additional 3-4 minutes.
5) Remove chicken from skillet and drain excess fat. I like to set the chicken on a paper plate for easier cleanup.
6) Add remaining butter to skillet. Add garlic and cook until fragrant.
7) Add cream, broth, lemon juice, thyme, and Parmesan. Stir and bring to a boil.
8) Boil for 3-5 minutes until slightly thickened. Add greens and cook until wilted.
9) Return chicken to pan (or, if using a baking dish, place chicken in sprayed baking dish and pour sauce/greens over the top.
10) Bake for 35-30 minutes or until chicken reaches 165 degrees on the inside.
11) Enjoy! Serve with garlic mashed cauliflower or cauliflower and radishes to sop up the yummy sauce.

4 servings

<u>Nutrition:</u>
Calories: 278
Carbs: 2.6g
Fiber: 0.6g
Net carbs: 2g
Protein: 15.9g
Fat: 22.7g

No Sugar Added Marinara Sauce

Ingredients

1 28-ounce can of San Marzano Certified Tomatoes
¼ can of water
2 cloves minced garlic
1 T olive oil
1 tsp red pepper flakes
1 tsp salt
1 tsp erythritol (optional)
1 T onion powder
1 tsp Italian seasoning
7-8 fresh basil leaves OR 1 tsp dried basil.

Instructions

1) Heat olive oil in large saucepan over low-medium heat.
2) Add garlic and red pepper flakes. Stir and cook until fragrant, then set aside and turn the burner off.

3) Pour tomatoes with their juice into a medium-sized bowl.

4) With clean hands, mash the tomatoes until they are pulpy.

5) Carefully add tomatoes to saucepan. Fill the empty can ¼ of the way full with water and add water.

6) Add erythritol, onion, salt, and Italian seasoning.

7) Stir to combine. Return to heat and cook on low for 30 minutes.

8) Add basil. Cover and simmer for 10 additional minutes.

9) If using fresh basil, pluck out fresh basil leaves.

10) If desired, blend until smooth. For a chunkier sauce, leave as is.

7 servings, about ½ cup each.

Nutrition:
Calories: 30
Carbs: 6g
Fiber: 3g
Net carbs: 3g
Protein: 1g
Fat: 2g.

No-Pasta Lasagna

Ingredients

3 medium zucchini
3 cups mozzarella cheese
1 cup Parmesan cheese

1 lb 80-85% lean ground beef
1 clove garlic
1 t onion powder
¼ tsp salt
Additional salt and pepper to taste
Additional mozzarella for the top
1 batch no-sugar-added marinara sauce OR 1 jar low-carb spaghetti sauce

Instructions

1) Preheat oven to 400° F.
2) Spray 8x8 baking dish with cooking spray
3) Wash zucchini and cut lengthwise into long, thin slices. A mandoline slicer would work great for this, but a sharp knife also works.
4) Lay zucchini out on clean tea towel or paper towels. Sprinkle with ¼ tsp salt. Set aside.
5) In a medium bowl, combine mozzarella and parmesan.
6) Brown the ground beef in a skillet over medium heat.
7) Add garlic and onion, salt and pepper to the ground beef and cook until garlic is fragrant.
8) Add sauce to ground beef mixture and stir. Reserve ½ cup sauce for the top of the lasagna.
9) Ladle about 1 cup of the sauce mixture into the bottom of the baking dish. Add a layer of zucchini slices.
10) Add a layer of the mixed shredded cheese.
11) Repeat until out of ingredients. Top with the reserved half cup of sauce mixture and sprinkle with additional mozzarella.

12)   Bake for 30-40 minutes or until cheese on top is golden brown and the middle of the lasagna is bubbling.

13)   Let rest for 5-10 minutes and then enjoy.

<u>Nutrition:</u> (without sauce. Add sauce used to the recipe and calculate for an accurate count).
Calories: 257
Carbs: 5g
Fiber: 1g
Net carbs: 4g
Protein: 23g
Fat: 16g

Rosemary Garlic Pork Chops

Ingredients

4 bone-in pork chops weighing about 2 pounds total
4-6 sprigs fresh rosemary or 1 T dried rosemary
3-4 cloves minced garlic
½ tsp white pepper
½ tsp black pepper
½ tsp salt, or to taste
2 T olive oil
1 cup water

Instructions

1) In a large skillet with a lid, heat olive oil over medium heat

2) Season pork chops with salt, black pepper, and white pepper. Be sure to get both sides.
3) Sear pork chops in a hot pan for 3-4 minutes. Flip and sear the other side.
4) Add water, rosemary, and garlic. Stir and bring to a boil.
5) Cover and reduce heat to low. Simmer until water has evaporated, about 10-20 minutes.
6) Serve with asparagus gratin, roasted cauliflower, and radishes, or another delicious side dish.

4 servings

<u>Nutrition:</u>
Calories: 277
Carbs: 1g
Fiber: 0g
Net carbs: 1g
Protein: 26g
Fat: 18g

For the next 4 recipes, you will need a vegetable spiralizer or pre-spiralized zucchini noodles. The spiralizer is available in home and kitchen stores and online, while many grocery stores have pre-spiralized zoodles in the produce section.

Zoodles Alfredo

Ingredients

2 pounds fresh zucchini - or 2 pounds zucchini noodles
1 cup heavy cream
2 cups freshly grated parmesan cheese
½ stick butter
2 cloves minced garlic
1 tsp freshly ground black pepper
Salt to taste
Toppings like cooked chicken, bacon, shrimp, sausage (optional; not included in nutrition calculations.)
Instructions

1) Spiralized zoodles according to spiralizer's instructions.
2) Place zoodles in a colander in the sink and sprinkle with ¼ tsp salt.
3) Meanwhile, melt butter in a medium-to-large skillet over medium heat. When foaming, add garlic.
4) Cook until garlic is fragrant, 1-2 minutes.
5) Add cream and whisk to combine. Turn heat down to medium-low.
6) While whisking, add pepper and grated parmesan. Whisk until sauce is smooth and creamy.
7) Keep sauce, hot over medium-low heat, but do not allow to boil. Stir often.
8) Squeeze zucchini noodles to get out extra water. To make this easier, you can pour them into a tea towel and squeeze the towel out over the sink.

9) Add squeezed zucchini noodles to the sauce, tossing with tongs to combine.

10) If desired, top with cooked chicken, shrimp, or bacon and extra Parmesan cheese.

11) Serve and enjoy

6 servings

<u>Nutrition:</u>
Calories: 344
Carbs: 7g
Fiber: 1g
Net carbs: 6g
Protein: 13g
Fat: 30g

Zoodles with Brown Butter

Ingredients

2 pounds zucchini (or 2 pounds zucchini noodles)
¼ tsp salt
½ stick butter
6-8 fresh sage leaves OR 1 tsp rubbed sage
½ cup freshly grated parmesan cheese
Freshly ground black pepper.

Equipment
Light-bottomed skillet or saucepan - you need to be able to see the butter changing colors

Instructions

1) Spiralize zucchini if not using pre-made zoodles. Place in a colander in the sink and sprinkle with the salt. Allow to sit while you make the sauce.
2) Melt the butter in the saucepan over low-medium heat.
3) Continue to cook the butter, stirring constantly, until it smells nutty and is light brown in color. This is easy to burn, so be sure to watch carefully.
4) Add sage to butter and stir well. Remove from heat.
5) Squeeze zucchini noodles to remove extra moisture. Placing them in a tea towel and squeezing the towel over the sink can make this easier.
6) Add zoodles to butter and return to heat. Toss to combine.
7) Serve into individual bowls and top with the Parmesan cheese and freshly ground black pepper. Enjoy!

4 servings

<u>Nutrition:</u>
Calories: 182
Carbs: 7g
Fiber: 2g
Net carbs: 5g
Protein: 7g
Fat: 15g

Zoodles Carbonara

Ingredients

2 pounds zucchini OR 2 pounds pre-made zoodles
¼ tsp salt
8 pieces of bacon
4 eggs plus 4 egg yolks (save the whites for something else)
4 cloves minced garlic
2 cups freshly grated parmesan cheese
Freshly ground black pepper

Instructions

1) Spiralize zucchini if not using pre-made zoodles. Place in sink and sprinkle with ¼ tsp salt.
2) Meanwhile, chop bacon into small pieces and render until crispy over low heat.
3) While bacon is cooking, beat eggs, egg yolks, and freshly ground pepper together until no streaks of white remain.
4) Remove bacon from skillet and place on paper towels to drain.
5) Add garlic to skillet with bacon grease and cook until fragrant.
6) Squeeze zucchini noodles to remove extra moisture. You can wrap them in a tea towel or paper towels to make this easier.
7) Add squeezed zucchini noodles to bacon grease and garlic and toss lightly to coat. Add half of cooked bacon and heat until zoodles are very hot.
8) Add parmesan cheese and toss to combine.

9) Remove from heat and pour in egg mixture, stirring constantly until eggs are just lightly cooked and create a creamy sauce.

10) Top with remaining bacon and serve with extra cheese and freshly ground pepper, if desired.

4 servings

<u>Nutrition:</u>
Calories: 415
Carbs: 6g
Fiber: 1g
Net carbs: 5g
Protein: 32g
Fat: 29g

Zoodles Marinara

Ingredients

2 pounds zucchini OR 2 pounds prepared zucchini noodles
¼ tsp salt
1 recipe no sugar added marinara sauce OR 1 jar of preferred low-sugar marinara sauce
1 T olive or coconut oil
2 cups mozzarella cheese

Instructions

1) Spiralize zucchini if not using pre-made zoodles. Place in a colander in the sink and sprinkle with ¼ tsp salt. Let sit for 10 minutes.
2) Squeeze moisture out of zucchini noodles. Using a tea towel or paper towel helps.
3) In a medium-to-large skillet, heat olive oil.
4) Add squeezed zoodles and stir.
5) Add sauce to skillet. Stir and cook until heated through.
6) Portion out into individual bowls, top evenly with cheese, and serve.

4 servings

<u>Nutrition:</u> (does not include marinara.)
Calories: 237
Carbs: 9g
Fiber: 2g
Net carbs: 7g
Protein: 17g
Fat: 15g

Keto Bread

In addition, of course, you cannot eat without bread. The Keto diet also provides the possibility of eating bread. Below are five recipes for cooking bread. However, for your training, I wrote the recipes without nutrition facts. Try to calculate them yourself

Almond Keto bread for any dish

Ingredients

1/4 cup pure almond flour
5 tablespoons finely chopped psyllium*
2 teaspoons baking powder
1 teaspoon sea salt
2 teaspoons vinegar (preferably apple cider)
1/4 cup of strong boiling water
3 egg whites
2 tablespoons sesame seeds (optional)

Instructions

1) Combine all dry ingredients; mix thoroughly.
2) Preheat oven to 350F.
3) Bring water to boil. Add egg whites and apple cider vinegar to dry ingredients. Mix all together with mixer for 30 seconds. Finish mixing only after the dough is ready for molding.
4) With wet hands, form 7-8 small portions of dough.
5) Lightly grease baking sheet with butter; also lightly cover the small portions of dough with butter. Sprinkle sesame seeds on each portion (optional).

6) Bake for approximately one hour until completely cooked. Determining when it is done is simple: Thump on the bottom of the bread with your thumb (like hitting a drum); if it is ready an empty hollow sound will be heard.

<u>Psyllium</u> or plantain flea is a leafy-stemmed Eurasian plantain. It is a cellulose and, in addition, a prebiotic. Psyllium is useful because it swells while in the intestine and helps to move the food. Natural laxative. Helps with constipation and diarrhea. Promotes the stabilization of blood sugar. Maintains healthy weight and normal cholesterol.

Keto bread with cheese

Ingredients

3 eggs
0.22 pounds of cream cheese
¼ tsp salt
½ tablespoon psyllium *powder*
½ teaspoon baking powder.

Instructions

1) Separate egg whites from egg yolks. Save egg yolks for later.
2) Whisk egg whites together with salt. Beat to a foam consistency, so that it does not fall out of the inverted container.

3) Mix yolks with cream cheese. Add psyllium and baking powder.
4) Carefully transfer whipped egg whites into a mixture made from yolks.
5) With wet hands, lay 7-8 small portions of dough on the dripping pan.
6) Bake in the middle of the oven at 350F for about 30 minutes. Bread should become golden in color.
7) Such bread can be used for rolls. You can combine with whipped cream and berries.

Paleo Bread from Flax

Ingredients

2 cups well-ground flax seeds
5 eggs
½ cup water
⅓ cup of melted cream or coconut oil
1 teaspoon soda
1 teaspoon apple cider vinegar
½ teaspoon sea salt
1 tablespoon sesame seeds.

Instructions

1) Thoroughly grind flax seeds in coffee grinder or food processor.
2) Whisk eggs with salt and water in one container.
3) Add crushed flex seeds, soda and vinegar to the beaten eggs. Mix everything thoroughly.

4) Pour in coconut or butter and bring to a homogeneous consistency.
5) Grease baking dish.
6) Transfer dough to baking dish.
7) Bake for 50-60 minutes at 350 ° F.

Keto Waffles from Flax

Ingredients

5 eggs (eggs can be replaced with 5 tablespoons of flax *powder*, adding 15 tablespoons of water)
½ cup boiled water or coconut milk
2 cups flax flour
a cup of coconut or butter
1 teaspoon soda
⅓ teaspoon sea salt

Instructions

1) Thoroughly grind flax in coffee grinder or food processor.
2) Whisk eggs while adding salt, and water or coconut milk.
3) Add flax flour and soda. Stir thoroughly. At the end, add oil.
4) Allow dough to stand for about 10 minutes.
5) Make waffles on the waffle maker.

Keto Buns

Ingredients

8 eggs
1.5 cups water
6 tablespoons melted butter
1 cup coconut flour
4 tablespoons psyllium
1 teaspoon soda
1 tablespoon apple cider vinegar
1 teaspoon sea salt
1 teaspoon garlic powder
Sesame *seeds* for sprinkling (optional)

Instructions

1) Preheat the oven to 350F.
2) Mix eggs, water and oil thoroughly.
3) Add salt and garlic. Then add coconut flour, psyllium, soda and vinegar. Stir to a homogeneous consistency.
4) Make small portions of dough.
5) Spread the portions on a baking sheet, sprinkle with sesame and bake for approximately 30 minutes.

Keto-Friendly Foods Nutrition Guide

*Information is taken from the United States Department of Agriculture's website. Always read your own nutrition labels for the best accuracy.

Food	Calories	Carbs (in grams)	Fiber (in grams)	Net Carbs (in grams)	Protein (in grams)	Fat (in grams)
Meats	-	-	-	-	-	-
Beef, ground, 85% lean, 1 lb	727	0	0	0	71	47
Beef, ground, 90% lean, 1 lb	685	0	0	0	73	41
Beef, chuck, 1 lb	990	0	0	0	78	73
Beef, corned, 1 lb	797	1	0	1	58	60
Beef, dried, 1 oz	43	0	0	0	9	.5

Chicken breast, skin-on, bone-in, 1 lb	572	0	0	0	86	23
Chicken leg, skin-on, bone-in, 1 lb	540	0	0	0	53	35
Chicken thigh, skin-on, bone-in, 1 lb	540	0	0	0	53	35
Mackerel, 1 lb	864	0	0	0	80	48
Pepperoni, full fat, 30g/16 slices	150	0	0	0	5	14
Pork, bacon, 1 lb	765	0	0	0	52	59
Pork, ribs, 1 lb	702	0	0	0	51	54

Pork, rinds, .5 ounces	80	0	0	0	9	5
Pork, shoulder, 1 lb	819	0	0	0	61	62
Salmon, 1 lb	651	0	0	0	98	26
Tuna, canned, water packed, 1 can (6.5 ounces)	144	0	0	0	32g	2g
Dairy	-	-	-	-	-	-
Butter (see fats)	-	-	-	-	-	-
Cheddar, shredded, 1 cup	455	4	0	4	28	37
Colby jack, shredded, 1 cup	434	4	0	4	27	22
Cottage cheese, full fat, 1	206	7	0	7	23	9

cup						
Cream cheese, full fat, 1 ounce	97	1	0	1	2	10
Heavy whipping cream, 1 T	51	0	0	0	0	6
Mozzarella, shredded, 1 cup	341	4	0	4	29	23
Neufchatel cheese, 1 ounce	57	1	0	1	2	4
Parmesan, grated, 1 cup	345	3	0	3	31	23
Provolone, sliced, 1 slice	100	1	0	1	7	8
Sour cream, full fat, 1 T	28	0	0	0	0	3

Fats	-	-	-	-	-	-
Bacon grease, 1 T	114	0	0	0	0	13
Butter, 1 T	100	0	0	0	0	12
Coconut oil, 1 T	117	0	0	0	0	14
Mayonnaise, 1 T	94	0	0	0	0	10
Vegetables						
Asparagus, 1 lb	91	18	10	8	10	1
Avocado, medium, whole	234	12	10	2	3	21
Broccoli, frozen, 1 cup	27	5	3	2	3	0
Cauliflower, 1 head, medium	147	29	12	17	11	2

Celery, 1 stalk, medium	6	1	1	0	0	0
Green beans, canned, 1 cup	34	6	3	3	2	0
Kale, 1 cup	33	6	2	4	3	1
Onion, green, 1 stalk	5	1	0	1	0	0
Radishes, 1 cup, sliced	19	4	2	2	1	0
Spinach, 3 cups	21	2	1	1	2	0
Zucchini, skin-on, 1 pound	73	13	4	9	5	1
Fruit	-	-	-	-	-	-
Blackberries, 1/4 cup	22	6	2	4	.5	0

Blueberries, ¼ cup	21	6	1	5	.5	0
Lemon, 1 medium	17	6	2	4	.5	0
Lime, 1 medium	20	7	2	5	.5	0
Raspberries, ¼ cup	16	4	2	2	.5	0
Strawberries, ¼ cup, halves	12	3	1	2	0	0
Nut & Seed Products	-	-	-	-	-	-
Almond butter 2 T	190	6	3	3	6	17
Almond flour, 1 cup	640	24	12	12	24	56
Almond meal, 1 cup	640	24	12	12	24	56

Almond milk, unsweetened, 1 cup	30	1	0	1	1	2.5
Almonds, 1 oz	164	6	4	2	6	14
Cashew milk, unsweetened, 1 cup	25	1	0	1	1	2
Cashews, 1 ounce	163	9	1	8	4	13
Chia seeds, 1 T	60	5	5	0	3	3
Coconut flour, 1 cup	480	64	40	24	16	16
Coconut, unsweetened, 1 oz	187	7	5	2	2	19
Flaxseed, ground, 1 T	55	3	3	0	2	4

Macadamia nuts, 1 oz	204	4	2	2	2	22
Peanut butter, unsweetened, natural, 2 T	191	6	2	4	7	16
Peanuts, 1 oz	161	5	2	3	7	14
Pecans, 1 oz	196	4	3	1	3	20
Walnuts, 1 oz	185	4	2	2	5	18

Conclusion

Well, we finished the examination of one of the most effective diets - keto diet. I hope the material provided helped you to get everything you need to create your personal keto diet of life style.

Of course, the topic of the ketogenic diet is very popular and constantly developing. It is not possible to disclose all aspects of this approach in this book. There are new scientific studies, and new developments and testimonies of those who have tried the keto diet in real life. Moreover, when you begin to practice it, you—yourself—will discover many new and interesting things.

The task of this book was not to provide you with all the material on this topic. The main thing was to prepare you to move from theory to practice. From reading to a real keto diet and life style. Now, it's up to you.

To summarize, I would like to give you some advice:

- If you have problems with your health, first get a medical examination. Keto diet is contraindicated for people with certain diseases.

- Carefully study the list of allowed products and create your own list that matches your culinary preferences.

- Be careful in planning. At this time, the restructuring of the body will begin and it will work in a slowed-down mode.

- Plan your time, so that you have enough for cooking.

- Do not forget to include green vegetables in your food! They are the source of fiber, which is necessary for normal operation of the intestine.

- Drink at least 8 glasses of clean water a day.

- Increase the use of cold-pressed coconut oil: it is a source of triglycerides of medium length, which easily turn into ketones.

- Do not limit your salt intake. Salt helps restore the electrolyte balance, which is disturbed by keto-diet.

- If you are doing sports, you need to know that your training potential may decrease because glycogen stores in muscles decrease on the keto diet.

Engage in moderate exercise—this is another very common piece of advice for people who follow a keto diet. Sports exercises in combination with keto diet produce an amazing effect.

In general, compliance with all the rules of the keto diet will lead you to desired results. Experience shows that a person can lose up to 3-4 pounds a week, depending on the body's individual characteristics.

Most importantly, in conclusion, I want to say that even the best diet will not be effective for you if you do not fulfill one simple condition. Be focused, and be ready to go through small, temporary difficulties while you live up to the new rules.

If you are ready to fulfill this condition, then after a couple of months on the keto diet you will see a unique effect with own eyes.

The Keto diet will open amazing results for you; you will get rid of excess weight and your life will be filled with happiness and health.

This is what I want you!

Lastly, dear friend, brother, sister, I would like to ask you one thing that I would appreciate very much! Respectfully, I ask you to leave a review about this book on the Amazon website.

Your review is very important to me for several reasons:
- First, it gives me information about how useful my book is and what other topics need to be described.
- Secondly, your appreciation of the book and your review will increase the chances that this book will be bought by other people.

So, I'm waiting for your evaluation and review! Thank you in advance!

To remind you, by buying this book and giving a review with high marks and positive feedback, you support:
- The work of the rehabilitation center for drug addicts, alcoholics and criminals.
- Charity ministry in two prisons.

- A future missionary trip to Indonesia (Kalimantan).